Oh, Thank God I Have Prostate Cancer!

A Patient's View

"been there, done that!"

HARVEY SILVER

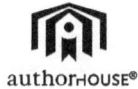

authorHOUSE®

*According to the American Cancer Society's Facts and Figures, it is estimated that in 2007 there will be 218,890 new cases of Prostate Cancer in the United States

AuthorHouse™
1663 Liberty Drive
Bloomington, IN 47403
www.authorhouse.com
Phone: 1-800-839-8640

First published by AuthorHouse 1/19/2011

ISBN: 978-1-4567-2165-7 (sc)
ISBN: 978-1-4567-2164-0 (e)

Library of Congress Control Number: 2011900072

Printed in the United States of America

Any people depicted in stock imagery provided by Thinkstock are models, and such images are being used for illustrative purposes only. Certain stock imagery © Thinkstock.

This book is printed on acid-free paper.

Forward by Dr. Bui

Prostate cancer is the most common cancer of men in the United States. It is the second leading cause of cancer death in the US. However, if caught early, prostate cancer is curable. Every day in my urology practice, I am faced with having to deliver this new diagnosis to many men. Oftentimes receiving the diagnosis of prostate cancer can cause significant distress. Most of the distress is related to not fully understanding the treatment options and what each option entails. Surgery is one of the options, which often stir significant uncertainty. Recent advancements in medical technology have made robotic surgery for prostate cancer safer, more precise and feasible.

There are very few publications available from a patient's perspective that may help others confronted with having to decide on surgical treatment. In this book, you will learn about one man's personal experience with da Vinci robotic assisted laparoscopic prostatectomy for the treatment of his prostate cancer.

The author presents a very humanizing perspective about his ordeal. The writing is very entertaining as well as informative. The author provides detailed accounts of his experience before, during and after his robotic prostatectomy. He provides practical insight and advice to those considering robotic prostate surgery. His hindsight perspective should provide consolation and confidence to others that full recovery is indeed possible following robotic prostate surgery.

Dr. Matthew Bui,

Director of Minimally Invasive and Robotic Surgery

Tower Urology

Cedars-Sinai Hospital.

Contents

INTRODUCTION

My name is Harvey Silver. I was 65 years young when I had my prostate removed. I had been tracking my PSA tests for 10 years as they fluctuated from 3.2 to 4.2. I had a biopsy ten years ago and it was negative. Then a few months ago, it went up to 6.0. Prior to the biopsy, the urologist did "a more thorough" digital exam and did feel something. I had a biopsy. My Gleason score was 6.

Maybe because I just assumed the biopsy was going to be positive, and assumed I was going to have to have surgery, I was almost relieved. And while I could have taken a more wait and see position, I made the decision to have surgery. I wanted it out and gone from my life.

I spent ten years worrying about it. I spent ten years wondering each time I got up at night to go to the bathroom if it was a strong stream, if this meant my prostate was enlarged, if this meant I had prostate cancer. So for me, the logic was simple. While I had a low Gleason, it was not going to go away on its own accord. The odds were that it was in its very early stages and still very localized in my prostate, and the words of my former internist rang in my ears. At one of my annual checkups he made the passing comment that prostate cancer was not a good way to die!

Many years earlier my father made me visit a family friend who was dying of prostate cancer. While forty years have passed, I can still see him lying in his bed, gaunt with his bright blue eyes looking at me while he squeezed my hand. The decision for me was an easy one.

Also, in the two years previous to this, I had six other close friends diagnosed with prostate cancer. Two chose to do the seeds, the others the traditional open surgery. All had very

different experiences and all are living and enjoying life. BUT...
and this is not a pitch for the robotic procedure, but... I chose
to go with the robot, and for me, it was as good an experience
as you can have. Trust me, I would have much rather spent a
couple of weeks in Hawaii, but that wasn't one of the surgical
options!

So, from me to you, here are a few things that I think you need
to keep in mind.

First, my experience won't be yours. Neither will anyone
else's.

Second, one of the interesting aspects of this process is that
you should absolutely talk to more than one physician, and
more specifically you should talk to different physicians who
advocate different approaches. One of the surgeons I met
with who advocated the traditional "open" procedure made the
comment that more than the process, the critical factor was the
skill of the physician. And I agree with that to an extent. I still
feel there are differences inherent to the processes.

I am not a doctor so I cannot give medical advice. The fact
is that there are circumstances and variables that impact
your options. For example, your age, Gleason score, size of
prostate, and other health variables all come into deciding the
right approach. There is not one correct answer. You must be
willing to go through the process, hopefully with a loved one,
collecting information. Then you will make the most informed
choice possible.

I say "with a loved one", because you will benefit from having
another set of ears listening. You should not be hesitant about
asking questions, particularly about your doctor's experience
and his results. Trust me the doctors you talk to will gladly
share with you this information and how good they are. Also be
prepared for them to ask you questions about your sex life. This
is an element of this operation, i.e. the ability to have erections
post surgery. So if this is going to be embarrassing in terms of

who is in the room with you, you need to be prepared for the questions, or simply tell the doctor that you would like to discuss this privately.

That said, this book is written about my experience and my experience is based on the procedure I chose. So you have to take this as an overview of what you may face and adapt it to your situation. Also, I have written this in very frank and candid terms; things men don't normally talk openly about, like how you clean yourself after having a BM when you have a catheter in! Well for that matter, having a good BM and the dynamics of the process.

So I hope this will be of value to you. I decided to try to write this thing while recuperating. There are lots of books available about prostate cancer, but nothing that approaches the subject from the patient's perspective... particularly after the surgery.

Thank you and good luck

Harvey Silver

PREFACE

"Oh thank God I have cancer!"

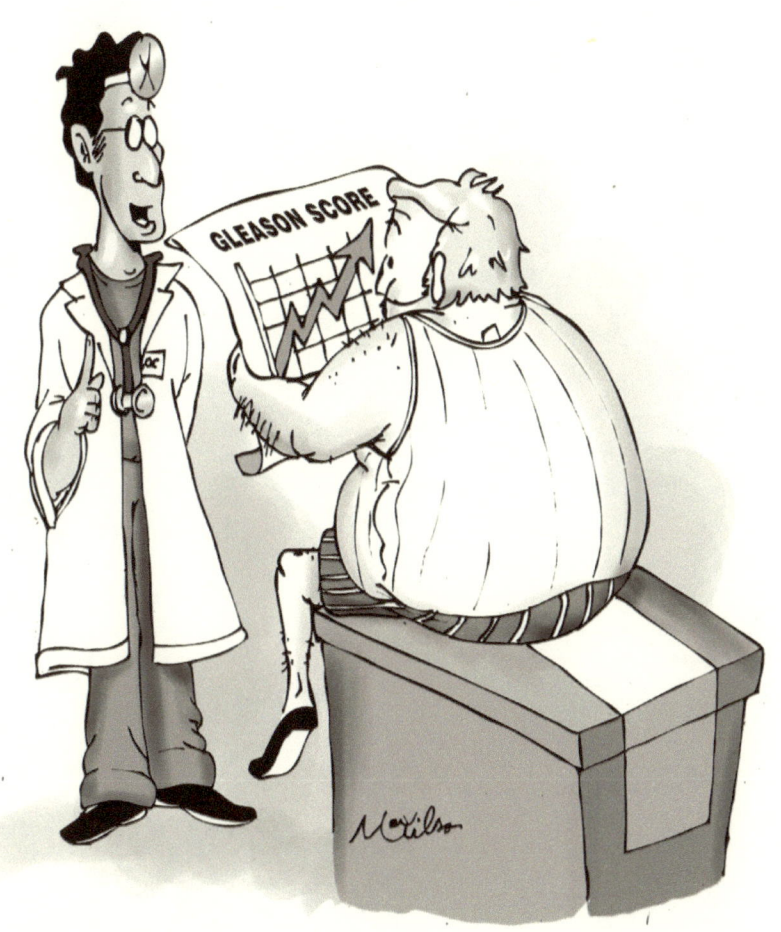

"...well, other than that, you are in great health!"

While talking to my doctor this morning, I was reminded that while each medical practice is going to have differences in their approach as well as in their process, the one thing that is common to all, is the emotional reaction of "getting the news".

I touch on some of the elements of the emotions and anxiety you may experience when "getting the news" in various places throughout the booklet. The odds are, however, if you are reading this, you have already gotten the news and hopefully have already begun to put this part of the process behind you.

I started this Preface with the subtitle, *"Oh thank God, I have cancer"*. I kind of meant it in this way: for many men, like me, the final "diagnosis" did not come out of the blue. I had been monitoring my PSA levels for ten years. For ten years the damn number would go up and down. I had a biopsy ten years earlier. So for me there was an agony of, alright, let's get it over with already.

Now while I say this lightly, my wife continued right up to the "meeting" with the urologist after the biopsy results came in positive, believing that I would not have cancer. WRONNNGGG!

Now I am one of those persons, who is convinced if my plane goes down, I will be one of the survivors, and this was even before the TV program LOST existed. The fact is this: much of what you are about to deal with is simply between your ears. IT REALLY IS ALL ABOUT ATTITUDE.

The fact is your cancer is going to be what it is going to be. That does not mean you can't be scared silly, or have anxieties, or worried about ever having a really good erection again! Of course with TV adds telling you that your biggest problem may be a four-hour erection, you just have to take one step at a time.

My experience was that the operation was not a matter of pain, it was a more a matter of discomfort.

It was not a matter of urinary incontinence, it was more a matter of how much time would be needed to regain full control

It is not a matter of if you will get an erection again, it will be a matter of time. And perhaps a little help from some pills, or other ingenious things they will show you.

Being diagnosed with prostate cancer IS NOT THE END OF THE WORLD. You will get through it. You are going to be amazed when you begin finding out how many people you know have gone through this. So you are not alone but your experience will be yours and no one else's. Keep a diary; talk to others about your experience and their experiences.

So enjoy the experience, milk it for all it is worth. Allow people to treat you nicely. Tell your wife that you really need to watch football all day on Sunday.

<u>And a special thanks to:</u>

First and foremost, I need to thank my wife of 42+ years, Susan. If I was ever difficult to live with, going through an experience like this raises the bar way high. As usual, she cleared it with room to spare.

And if you have children, no matter how good or how bad your relationship with them is, fathers occupy a unique space in everyone's life. And while everyone is going to reassure you, that all is going to be ok (which it probably will be), there is an unspoken anxiety that will exist, so be aware of this. You are not the only person having to cope with the scare of CANCER.

A special thanks to my children Michael, Claire, and son-in-law John who provided reassurances, both funny and serious when needed and spent many hours being my editor.

Then there are my friends who shared their experiences with prostate cancer: John D, Bill G, Dave M, Bill S, Jerry S, Cy Y, and Bob R.

I also want to acknowledge the illustrator, Mark Wilson. I think the addition of his artistic humor is terrific. You can view more of his work at: http://www.markseanwilson.com/

And lastly, a special thank to Dr Bui. His quiet but reassuring professionalism made this experience a whole lot easier.

THANK YOU.

CHAPTER 1.

PRE-SURGERY PREP

"Doing shots, liquid diets, not eating for 48 hours and other fun things"

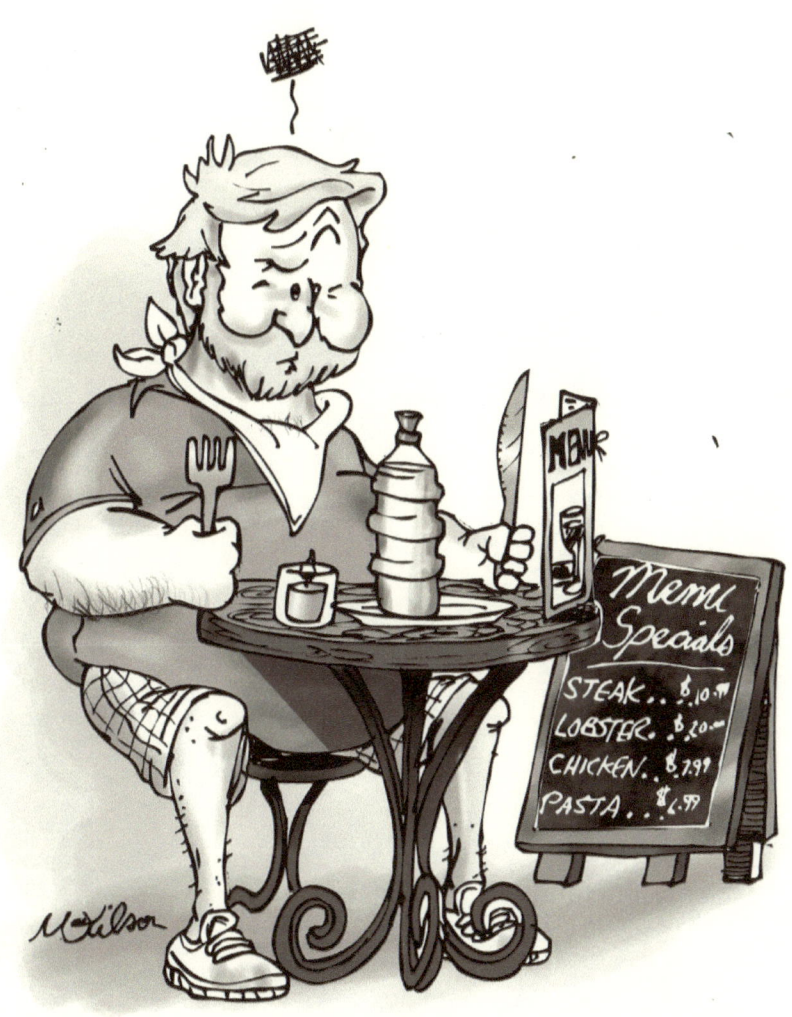

1

In mentally preparing for the surgery, there were two primary issues I kept agonizing over. One was the "prep" itself and the other "the catheter". More about the catheter in Chapter 2. Let's talk about the preparation,

Two elements about "the prep" concerned me. The first was not eating for almost 24 hours and the second was the dreaded enema.

My surgery was scheduled for 4:30 in the afternoon on a Thursday. My prep instructions had me going on a liquid diet starting on Tuesday afternoon and then not being able to drink anything after midnight before the operation.

I had never been on a liquid diet (which included jello) and could not imagine how this was going to work. Normally, when I did not eat for any length of time, I would not feel well, and sometimes got dizzy. I assumed this was from low blood sugar or something like that.

So, I went to the store and bought a variety of different energy drinks, for which I had never shopped. I also bought a variety of fruit drinks. One turned out to be particularly useful when I had to do the Fleet Enema Drink, but more on that later in this chapter.

Now I will admit that I did cheat a bit, but I did way better in terms of sticking to this than I ever imagined I would. Generally speaking, I am not very good about following orders. On Wednesday, the day before my surgery, I had an important business lunch meeting that I had scheduled and had forgotten about it in terms of "the prep." Not wanting to focus the meeting on my upcoming surgery, I had to eat something, right? I ordered a bowl of tomato soup while my colleague ate this fantastic looking lobster cob salad. Cheating just a little bit more, I added crackers to my soup. Hey, you can't eat tomato soup without crackers!

My wife made me a selection of different jello flavors. This was great, but I dare you to close your eyes and try to tell each flavor apart. They all taste the same!

Now for the good news: I was amazed at how easy the liquid diet was, except for that darn lunch meeting. For the most part, I really did just "eat" my drinks and jello. I drank as much as I wanted, and, because of the high carbohydrates in the energy drinks, I really was not hungry. I do suggest you store your drinks away from other foods, however, so that you won't be tempted like me, every time you open the refrigerator to get juice to drink.

Perhaps because I had not eaten, but more likely due to a high level of anxiety about the surgery, when I got to the hospital around 11:00 am on Thursday, I did not feel hungry or at least I didn't care about eating right then. I was thirsty, however. When I asked for some water, I got a sponge lollipop that lasted about two nano seconds. But that was long enough to get me on the gurney and into surgery. By that time, I was no longer thinking about food!

I encountered an issue during "the prep," which may or may not be common. Due to not eating, my enema (hang on, I'm getting to this), and the energy drink diet, I was actually dehydrated. This made finding my veins for the various needles more difficult.

When I was in college I had worked in a hospital drawing blood so I had some experience in the field, and was not happy at the thought of having them "hunt" for a vein. But here I was introduced to something new, which I told the technician was not necessary based on my college experience 45 years ago. I was offered a small local anesthesia injected into the site where they were going to put the IV. I declined initially not realizing that my veins had actually shrunk. After not finding the vein the first time – ouch – I acquiesced to the local anesthesia and am very happy I did. Otherwise, I think the hunt may still be going on.

The needle for the local was so small I really did not even feel it. Once that anesthesia was in place, they could probe all they wanted. I felt nothing and, I think, the technician's anxiety lessoned. Believe it or not, from my experience drawing blood, missing a vein and causing a person more pain and discomfort does cause anxiety for the person doing the probing!

So, I have now covered the first part of "the prep". Now on to the really fun part: THE ENEMA!

If you have ever had a colonoscopy or similar procedure you have already experienced the fun of a Fleet enema. The worst part I think is the drinking of the potion! When I went to buy mine at the drug store, I found that it came in two varieties, flavor (ginger lemon) and no flavor. Now the natural tendency is to go the flavor route. Then I began wondering how yucky would ginger lemon be? So I asked the pharmacist her opinion. First she said, go with the unflavored. Second, she gave me what turned out to be the best advice I could have gotten. The thing comes in a little 1 ½ oz bottle. The instructions tell you to mix it with 8 ounces of fruit juice, which means now instead of having to drink 1½ oz of really really really terrible stuff, you have to drink 8 ounces of really terrible stuff! So what she recommended was to drink the 1½ oz as a shot! It couldn't be worse than ouzo, a traditional Greek drink I've sampled in my past. I followed her advice with one small modification. Remember when I mentioned buying fruit drinks? Well one of the drinks I bought was a pineapple-coconut drink (think pina collada). It turned out to be kind of thick and syrupy. I poured the 1½ oz of Fleet into a small tumbler and mixed a very little amount of my fruit drink keeping the total volume small so that I could still do it as a shot. Once I did the shot, I followed it with a fruit juice chaser, water, and any other liquid I could get my hands on. You will want to drink lots of liquids because, trust me, everything will soon be leaving your body at a rapid rate, and will continue to do so for many hours.

My prep instructions had me doing the Fleet's thing twice, about an hour apart, after which you need to be prepared to spend some quality time in the bathroom. But BEFORE I got totally into this part of the procedure, I applied a generous portion of

5

petroleum jelly to my rectum. Also, I applied more after each of the many times I went to the bathroom. Finally, I found doing the "the paper work" immediately and often helped minimize the inevitable sore rear end.

Ok, so I made it through my two biggest prep concerns, the not eating and the enema, and neither of them turned out to be a big deal. It was time to let the surgeon go to work. Let's get on the table and get the show going!

CHAPTER 2.

WAKING UP…

"That's it… oh sxx!@#$%

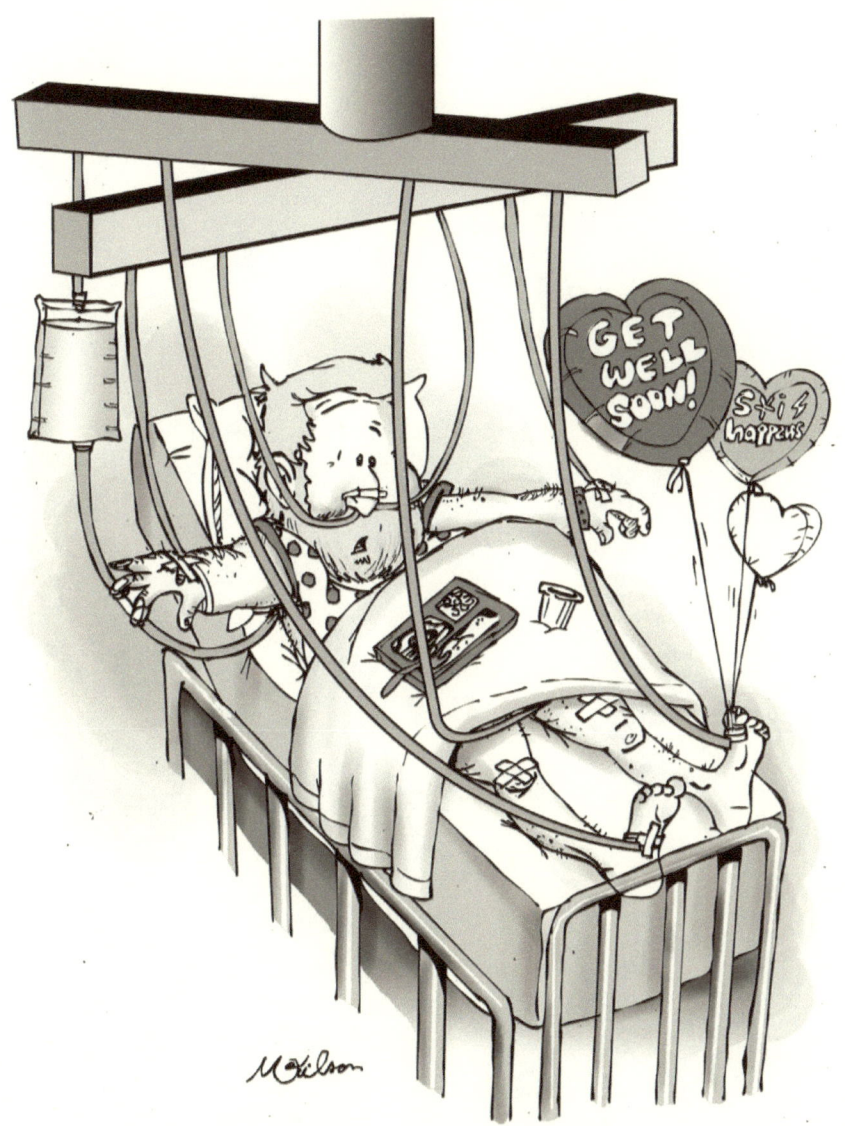

Well, they rolled me into the surgical suite and introduced me to *da Vinci:* the robot. That is about the last thing I remember. Then I woke up. I didn't really sense anything at this point, maybe a little disorientation, but someone in the room said it was a successful operation and all went well. I should also make mention that after they took out my prostate, they also repaired a hernia!

It wasn't long before they told me that they were going to take me to my room. When we got there they pulled the cart up next to the bed and told me to scoot over!

My reaction was like WHAT??? Are you crazy, I just had surgery? (I may have said a few other words, but we'll just leave it at that.) But they assured me that I could do this. And I did! It is not so much that I was in pain as much as I anticipated I would be. I felt weird feelings in my gut, probably due to seeing the tubes and things hanging on gizmos next to me. I had one of those little scopes with graphs and numbers blinking. It is like in the movies, except now you are the movie star!

Well, I successfully got into the bed. It wasn't as difficult as I feared.

At this point it was about 7:30pm, over 8 hours since I arrived at the hospital. In other words, it had been a very long day. Soon after, my wife and son (and his girlfriend) came into the room. They all seemed happy. I can't say the thought didn't cross my mind that they might know something bad that I hadn't yet been told and were just being brave. We visited for a while and then they left. I imagined they probably went to have a good dinner.

What came next was a long, long night.

Now I don't know how other hospitals work, but I have come to understand that in modern medicine pain management is now something that focuses on not having pain. The nurse came in and asked me if I was aware of the hospitals pain management grading system. I said no. She said that pain was graded on a scale from 1 (no pain) to 10 (lots of really really bad pain). This made sense, I guess. Then she said that when I got to about a 4 level, I should ask for pain pills. My immediate reaction, was something like what the hell constitutes a 4 level pain? Her answer was brilliantly simple. She said that when the pain got to a point where I felt I needed a pill that was a four level. I think that's what you call circular logic, but maybe I was still a little groggy. She never did tell me what happened at the 5 and beyond levels, and I didn't really want to know.

Honestly the pain wasn't that bad, but the comfort level sucked! I had a little gizmo on my finger measuring my blood oxygen. I had a drain tube coming out my side. I also had a catheter and an IV. Oh, yeah, I almost forgot, I also had seven little holes in my abdominal wall. Normally it's five holes, but because I also had a hernia fixed, I had two more holes.

I was in a private room so I could watch TV. I decided that I would try to stay awake watching TV as long as I could, so that I could pass out like I normally did every night on the couch before my wife woke me up to go to bed.

This kind of worked. While I was not hungry, I was thirsty and was able to have water. Do you know how good water really tastes? I can tell you, really really good! And I watched TV, and I did more or less fall asleep, for a little while at least. Unfortunately, next to the TV was a BIG clock... and it seemed to run very slowly. Time stands still when you're having fun!

Somewhere in the course of the night I decided I had reached pain level four. So I called for the nurse and eventually she showed up with a vicodin. Now, I have to admit, I had never taken one of these babies before, and I remembered my wife saying how some pain pills made her really dizzy. But I figured what the hell, I was bored and figured that I might as well try one of the puppies out. So I did.

Frankly, I have no idea if they helped or not. But I do believe that I tried a second one in the early hours of the morning.

While I am not sure if they helped, they didn't seem to have any negative effects on me, but I quit while I was ahead and did not ask for more.

Finally daylight came. By this time, I just wanted up. It just seems like all the bed sheets were jumbled up under me; I couldn't get comfortable; I really wanted to move my body. So I called the nurse. Pretty soon a gentleman came into my room to help me sit up, gave me a little cleaning up; and put these white spandex hose on my legs. They felt pretty good, at first.

Now came the challenge of getting up out of bed, tubes and all. I have to admit, that I was a bit apprehensive and didn't know if I was I going to be in pain; was I going to be dizzy; were my legs going to do their thing? Heck, I hadn't eaten for what seemed days and had been lying down for a day and a half.

I was also feeling really gassy, so I had another motivation for wanting to move. I hoped the simple act of walking would get my bowels going, which should relieve the gas.

I was a bit weak at first and unsure what I could really do. But to put this into a bigger perspective according to the doctor (it was just about 9 am) by 4:30 pm that same day I could go home if all was well. This meant walking to the car; and walking up steps in my house. So, while those first few steps were a little shaky, in retrospect, the process goes pretty quickly.

In fact, I knew that I would not be allowed to leave that hospital unless I was able to walk and that the act of walking was going to get my bowels moving, and that was going to help me get rid of the gas that was still in my gut. So I was motivated to walk.

After the short walk, I began thinking about food. At first they said nothing but clear liquids and jello and some soda crackers. Hey, didn't I already do this diet for several days before the surgery? But then a woman showed up and said I could be on a regular diet and gave me all kinds of things to choose from. I think they knew that once I tasted the hospital food, I wouldn't want to eat it. They were pretty much right.

Around noon, my wife and son showed up, coincidentally along with my food tray. I was amazed at how not interested in food I was. I thought I really wanted to eat, but it turned out that wasn't the case. And it was unappetizing enough that neither my wife nor son wanted to eat it either!

Somewhere in the next few hours, which I spent in a chair – I just didn't want to get back into that bed – the nurses began taking things out and off of me. A doctor visited and said I was doing great. Later my surgeon came in and said that I could go home later that afternoon. They took the IV out, the blood oxygen monitor, and then the biggie, the drain tube.

I had heard about this and was not looking forward to it. I had this long plastic tube somewhere inside my body and he was going to pull it out. It's one thing to see something like that on TV or hear someone tell you about it, but when the doctor is standing beside you – well, let's just say that while I normally like to watch these things, I turned my head and did not look. I think he gave me some instructions or something, but I don't remember. I do remember kind of a funny feeling, kind of like a mild burning sensation, and then it was out. Heh, no big deal.

So now all I had left was my catheter. I was told a nurse would come in and give me instructions on how to care for this and to change and empty bags, etc. And she did. It seemed pretty straightforward. More on this later.

OK, so now it was later in the afternoon, just about 24 hours since the surgery and I was ready to go home. I really wanted out of the hospital even though I really had an easy time of it all and nothing really to complain about regarding my stay. But, it's still a hospital and home is just better.

I got dressed in some Bermuda shorts wearing my leg bag. I was given two types of bags for the cath to drain into. One is a larger bag with about 2 liter capacity and the other a "leg" bag of about 500 cc capacity. The cath tube protrudes from your penis for about 10-12 inches. The end of this tube is then connected to the bag's tube. The leg bag simply is fastened to your leg by an upper and lower rubber band of sorts, like the rubber bands used in tourniquets when they draw your blood, but with little buttons for adjustments. I will talk more about this later. For now, just know that you are going home with this little guy strapped to your leg or you will be carrying the larger bag.

I got to the car and only would sit in the back seat, as the next to last thing I wanted was a seat belt around me. The very last thing I wanted was a seat belt around my gut *and* to have an accident. I envisioned an air bag exploding in my chest and abdomen. Normally I am a pretty assertive driver, but I found all I wanted was slow and easy. We got home in one piece, and thus began the next stage of this little adventure.

Chapter 3.

GAS GAS GAS PAIN PAIN PAIN

"And my shoulder hurts because...?"

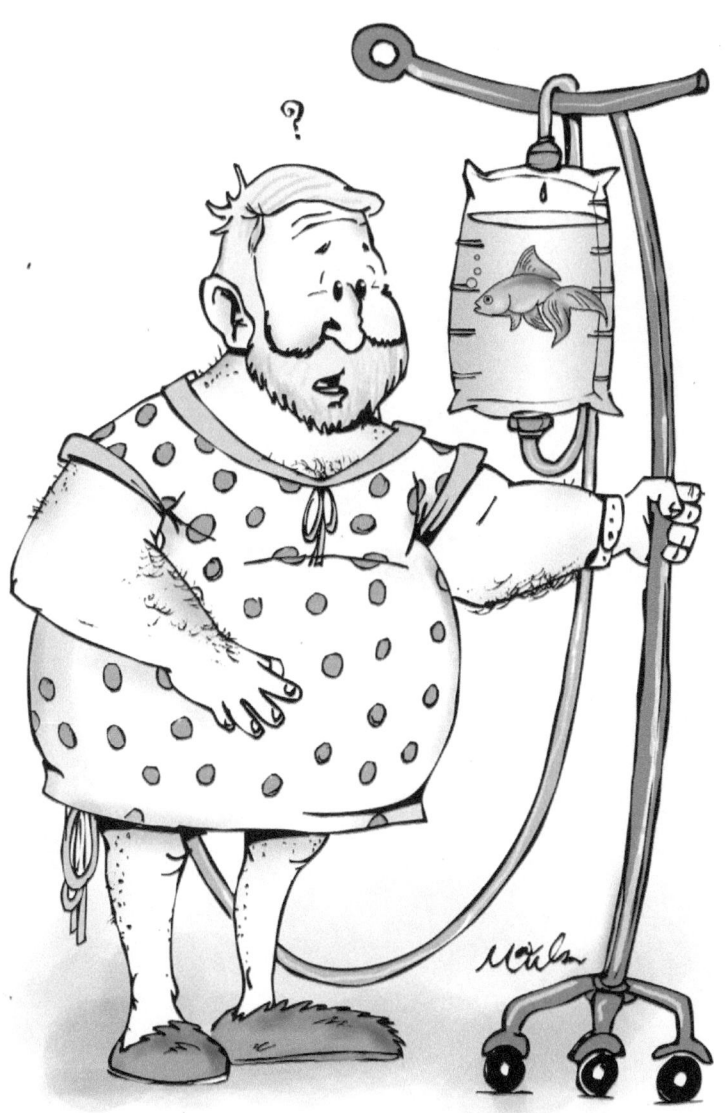

Ok, so I said in the introduction that this is all based on MY experience and that your experience will be different. Here is one of those areas, particularly if you did not have the *da Vinci* procedure.

When doing arthroscopic surgery, it is my understanding that they fill your abdominal cavity with CO_2 gas. This does a couple of things. First it pushes the organs away from the field of vision thereby giving the surgeon a better and cleaner view of the operating area. It also puts pressure on the surrounding tissues which results in less blood loss.

However, what goes in must come out. While they do everything they can to pull out as much gas as possible when the surgery is done, it does not all come out. This is like in a colonoscopy, if you have had that experience. Now eventually, within a couple of days of the surgery, the gas will be absorbed into your tissues, expelled, etc.

For me this took two days, but the day after surgery I experienced quite a bit of discomfort and pain in my right shoulder. In fact this was about the most significant pain I experienced in the entire procedure. What I found out is that the pain was being caused by the gas that was pressing on my diaphragm which pressed on a nerve which was manifested by the pain in my shoulder. Rubbing did not help; pills did not really help either.

One of the benchmarks you aim for post surgery is the passing of gas… the old fashioned way, not through your shoulder! For me it took almost 48 hours for this to happen. By late afternoon on Saturday (recall my surgery was on Thursday late afternoon) I was really uncomfortable, in fact, I was in so much pain that I called the doctor.

My abdomen felt really extended and bloated. I just wanted to put a pin in it to burst the balloon, so to speak. The doctor's words were essentially, be patient, it will pass. In the mean time I found myself pacing up and down waiting for the blessed event.

Thirty five years earlier, my wife was pregnant. Like most young parents to be, we went to Lamaze classes. In those classes I learned about "effleurage" – the gentle stroking of her abdomen while telling her she would soon feel better (while she told me something else I won't print here)! Well, guess what, effleurage works! So while I paced up and down, I gently rubbed my abdomen, while my wife said, "Now you know what it feels like!" I think she secretly enjoyed seeing me in a pregnant like state.

I am happy to tell you the doctor was right. Late that afternoon the dam broke and the gas began coming out. When it did, my shoulder pain went away with the gas!

At the beginning of this section, I again reinforced the "uniqueness" of each person's experience. Just a week ago, a close friend went through this same procedure, but at a different institution. Their procedure had some differences as well. When he told them about my shoulder pain experience, they were quite surprised and said this was quite rare. My friend had none of it!

However, another friend told me that I should write more about the pain (gas) he experienced. He found that walking up and down stairs slowly seemed to help more than just pacing back and forth. He too found that within forty eight hours of the operation, he began getting rid of the gas and felt almost instant relief.

I hope your experience will be more like my first friend's. But in case it is like mine, while doing effleurage, just keep telling yourself to be patient and that it will pass - literally.

Let's talk about pain in general. First there was not a lot of pain. I found it more of a matter of discomfort and anticipation of pain. Once I left the hospital, even though the doctor did give me a prescription for drugs, I never had it filled and only relied on over the counter pain pills. Your doctor will give you advice on what to take and how much. I will touch on sleep aids a bit later.

You need to get into your head that you are not going to break or tear open anything if you move about. I would suggest that you gingerly move around and see for yourself what your limits are. You may be pleasantly surprised by how much mobility you will have once you get over being scared to move around.

There were "other pains" that I also experienced, but they really weren't as much a pain as sensitivity, like a bruise. Unlike a bruise, however, these sensitivities were *inside* me. One was in the colon and the other was where I assume the anastomosis was – where the two ends of the urethra were joined i.e. pulled together. All I can say is that this seems to be a common thing and it went away as the tissues heal. One day you will go to the bathroom and realize that you had no other sensations or feelings that were different from the good old days, but it will take some weeks before this happens.

Chapter 4.

The Catheter

It's ok to touch your penis...

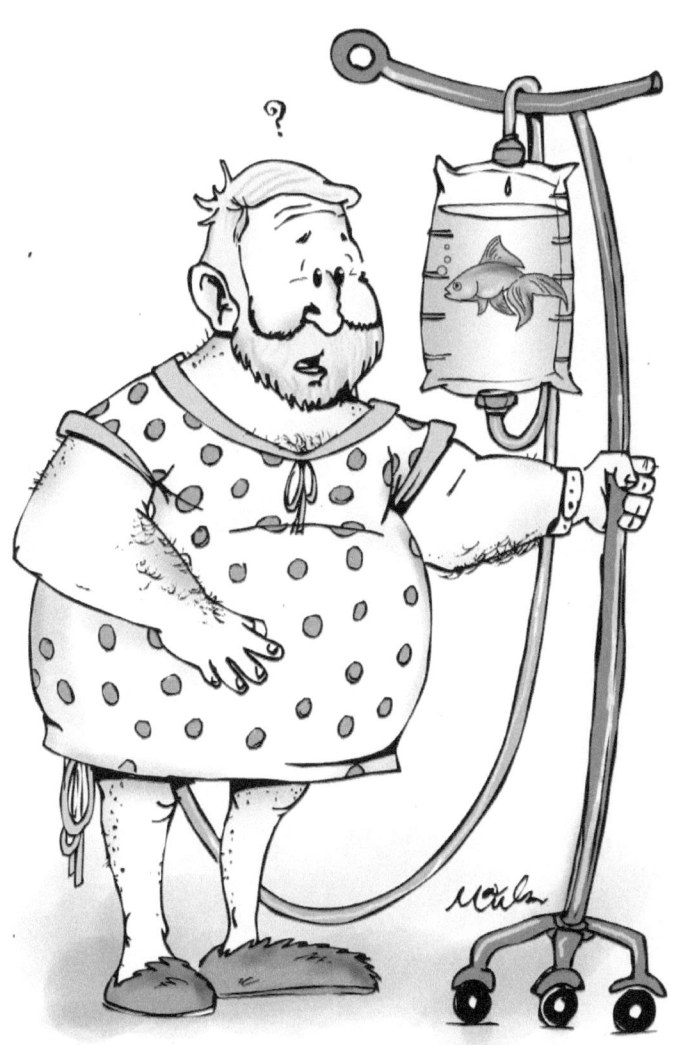

Before I left the hospital a person came into my room to give me instructions on how to care for the catheter and the "bag." I and everyone I've talked to were given two different bags, a big one and a small one I could wear on my leg, simply called "the leg bag."

The catheter tubing stuck out of my penis by about a foot. They showed me how to disconnect the bag and switch bags. They also showed me how to empty the bags. Needless to say I was worried about all of this, particularly about accidentally pulling the catheter out during the week I would have to wear it.

I worried about irritating my penis where the catheter came out by moving or touching it. I was worried about infection and cleanliness. I was told something about keeping the opening of my penis clean and to keep "crust" from forming at the point where the catheter comes out. That alone scared me. What the heck is crust doing around my penis?! In short I was nervous, concerned, and scared, but since they were telling me all this as I was trying to get out of the hospital, I didn't care. I just wanted to get home.

Now I can pretty much promise you that you will not remember exactly what you were told to do or how to do it. However, I can also pretty much assure you that it is not complicated nor that difficult.

So I went home and once there decided that I would use the leg bag. Unfortunately, I discovered that the little Velcro strap to hold the tubing snugly against my leg did not find its way into the goodie bag they gave me. Not to worry, I found an old elastic bandage and just cut it down and tied it to my leg, securing the tube. Every time I jiggled the tube – and my penis – I would freeze and hold my breath wondering if anything bad was going to happen. Nothing ever did!

Ok, so back to catheter and bag basics 101. My biggest concern, and that of my friends and others I have spoken with, is living with the catheter for a whole week. I am going to take the suspense out and jump to the bottom line: you will find this almost a non-issue and you will acclimate to the process pretty quickly. I easily customized and adapted and you will, too.

There are several elements to this subject: 1) Touching and moving the tube and your penis; 2) Changing of the bags; and 3) Emptying the bags.

The catheter is not just simply a long tube they stuck into the penis and bladder. I believe the correct product term is that it is a Foley Catheter – I assume named after its inventor Dr. Foley? Check it out: http://en.wikipedia.org/wiki/Foley_catheter. The catheter is held in place by a little balloon at the end, which is inflated, meaning it isn't going anywhere! You can touch it or move it from right leg to left leg. You can wash yourself, change bags, empty bags, and nothing bad, or painful, is going to happen.

I personally got so "comfortable," if you can say that, with the leg bag, that the biggest problem was remembering it needed to be drained every couple of hours. In fact my friend who just went through this napped one day with his legs up on the couch and when he woke found the bag filled and because his leg was up on the couch, it was not draining his bladder. This was quickly cured by simply sitting up and draining the bag.

One of the things I found was perhaps why people used to say I was full of it! I was amazed at how much urine I passed. In fact I was beginning to think I must have like a supersized bladder to have held all this. Note, this issue comes back into play a bit later after the catheter is removed.

Let's talk leg bag technique and strategy. I found that the rubber bands that secure the bag did irritate my legs and pulled on my hair, so I would change the bag from one leg to the other. It will scoot up and down a bit, but you will easily work through this. However, I found which leg you had it on did come into play when you had a BM and had to do the essential paper work associated with this process.

This process requires some twisting of the torso. I found that immediately post surgery this twisting was not comfortable AND was affected by whether you are you right handed or left handed. Well depending on your answer, I found that it mattered which leg my bag was on, in terms of ease of access based on which hand you use. If you are not following this discussion, I think it will become very obvious to you very quickly. The point here is to think about this when the time comes. You will figure out what best works for you!

Moving on to bag management. Each morning I immediately switched from my big bag, which you must use at night because of its larger capacity. As an aside, you might just want to keep the big bag on all day. I have two friends that did this. One rigged up a bucket with a handle and the other a shopping bag. They simply put the bag into the bucket or shopping bag and carried that around with them. Remember, you probably are not going to leave the house for the week you are catheterized, so this may not be an issue at all. I found myself walking in our yard and around the house with no problems, carrying my bag. I will talk about sleeping a bit later.

Changing bags is not a big deal, and draining them is even less. At first I would loosen the bottom strap of the leg bag to give me more movement so I could make sure I was over the toilet. Later I just simply left it all strapped up and got myself next to the toilet bowl, pulled the plug and let it flow. It was quick and easy. The big bag is even easier because it has a drain hose. Urine is essentially a sterile fluid; so don't get concerned if you get some on your hands.

I was a bit cautious, to say the least, about my first shower. I made sure my wife was in earshot and I did not fully close the bathroom door. I had my leg bag on for the shower. As the sub-title for this chapter states, it is ok to touch your penis and wash it. Nothing bad will happen. In fact, I found the warm water soothing on my abdomen. After the shower I also applied a bit of petroleum jelly to the opening of the penis around the catheter tube. Once I had my first shower, I became very comfortable with the process.

Now I am going to touch on a very interesting subject that both I and my friend experienced, so I assume it must be somewhat common. Shortly after his surgery, we were talking and he said something to the effect that he had "imploded". I knew exactly what he was referring to. If feels like your penis is being pushed or pulled back into your body, akin to an English bulldog's face! In reality, I found this even more pronounced after the catheter was removed. I was reminded about a conversation I had with another friend who opted not to have a surgical solution to his prostate cancer. He asked me if I knew how they connected the two ends of the urethra after the prostate was removed.

Let me digress here for a second. I don't want to assume that everyone totally understands the surgical process and the anatomy as it relates to the surgery. I could not find a simple drawing for use here, so I will attempt to explain in layman's terms a key point to understand. In the simplest of terms you have a tube (the urethra) running from the bladder through your penis. The prostate is like a roundish clamshell surrounding that tube. When the prostate is removed, the two ends of the urethra are cut at either end of the prostate. Therefore, a key element of the surgery is to then connect the two ends, one coming from the bladder and the other going into your penis. This is called an *anastomosis (the surgical union of two hollow organs, e.g. blood vessels or parts of the intestine, to ensure continuity of the passageway).*

So guess what. When you join to ends together, you need to pull a bit on both of them to get them to meet. And yes, you may end up pulling in such a way that your penis is slightly shorter afterwards --Ergo, the implosion feeling, and possibly a somewhat "shorter" penis.

Approximately 8 days after my surgery, I went to the doctor's office for a checkup and to have my catheter removed. I was really really not looking forward to this at all. It turned out to be a bit more complex a procedure than I had imagined. Before and during the removal they do tests to make sure everything is healed inside and there are no leakages, etc. The bottom line is this: it was not that bad a process. Again, the anticipation was worse than the actual event, and it is over pretty quickly. The actual removal probably does not take 3 seconds.

Now that I have covered the basics of dealing with the catheter, I had to figure out what to wear with my extra attachments.

Chapter 5.

What to Wear…

Hanging bags and other accoutrements…

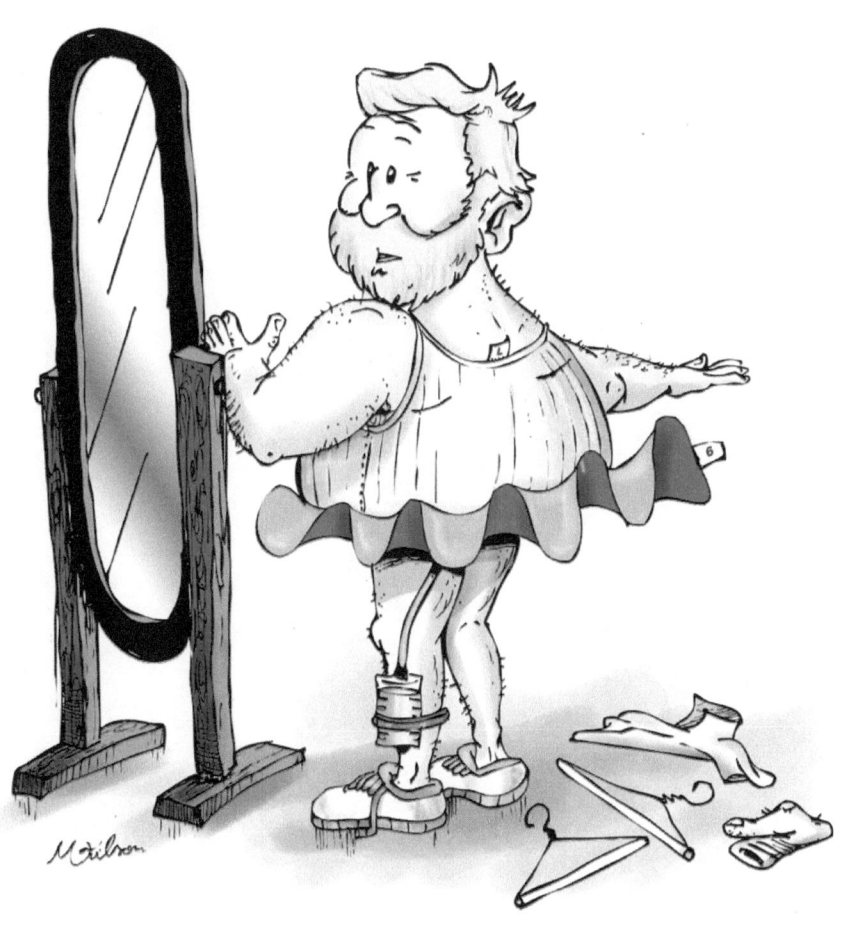

I have already touched on some of the issues of "the bags." Actually you will find this to be very straightforward. A key issue here will be time of year and climate you live in and other such things as whether you live in an apartment, condo building, or house with a yard, its degree of privacy, and your own comfort level with the issue of privacy and how people in your household may react to the sight of a "bag" filled with urine.

My surgery was done in August in Los Angeles, so outside temperatures were not a factor. I also live in a house with a yard, so I could wander around outside and be fairly private. At times, I just wandered about in my boxer shorts. And since it is very important that you walk a lot, these things do factor into the recuperation process.

I generally wore loose fitting Bermuda style shorts. Sometimes I did wear lounging pants that had very loose legs. A friend's wife found some old pants and cut out pockets, put in zippers, etc. The point is this: don't worry about this aspect of the procedure. If you are anything like me you are going to be concerned about how this all works with the catheter. Luckily, the answer is that it is not a big deal. But you should still think about it a little before the surgery so you can do a bit of planning. Of course there is always the bathrobe! You will have lots of options and will find things to wear and to be comfortable in at the same time. Also, keep in mind, you aren't going to be going out dancing and doing a lot of entertaining. Also, with a little bit of luck, you are going to get rid of the catheter in a week, like me. Plus, during that first week I was sore and tired, so I was not looking to go out much.

Chapter 6.

Sleeping

Yeah Right!!!

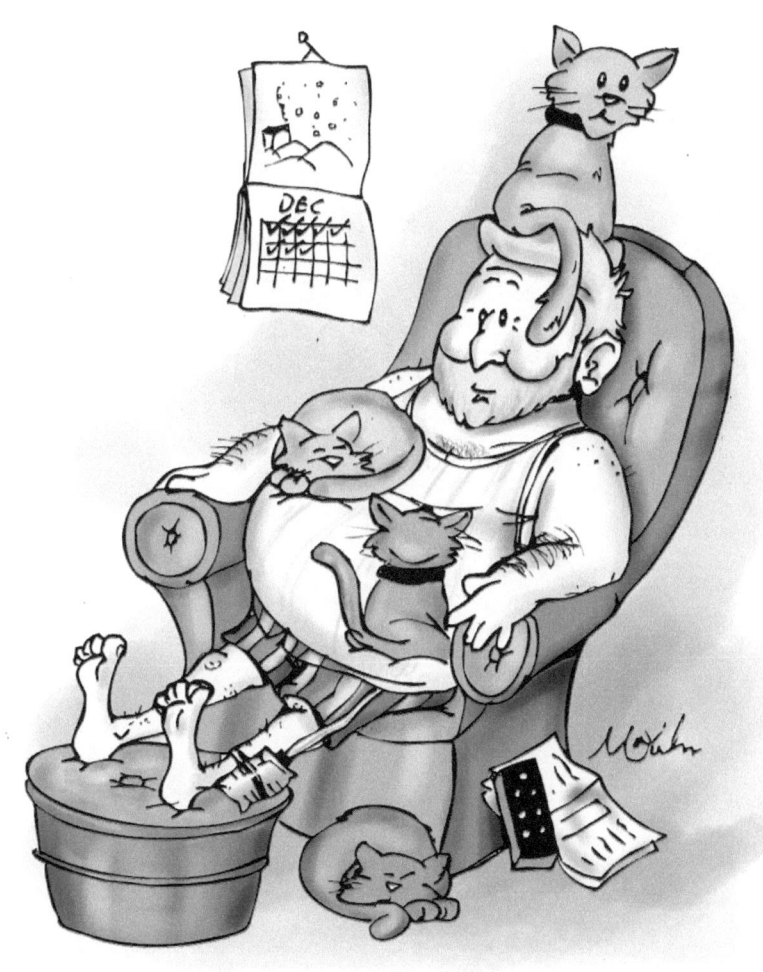

The only challenge I had sleeping was the first night after the surgery when I was in the hospital. It seemed like a forever night. I tried to stay awake and watch TV as long as possible. I just kept telling myself that it was just a matter of seven or eight hours that I had to get through. There is no rule that you have to sleep – you can wake, doze, sleep – just allow Mother Nature to take its course.

My hospital bed was cranked up not quite to a sitting position, but up more than is normal. Just get through the night. It will pass, trust me. Once morning came I began to get busy with nurse's aides, taking in some liquids, and help getting out of bed.

Once you get home you will be in your own space --but I did not say your own bed. The reason being, I found I was most comfortable sleeping in a recliner. My wife covered it with a sheet and gave me a couple of small pillows. I put one pillow in the small of my back and a light blanket to cover me. Before going to sleep, I put on the big bag. We put a towel on the floor, and the bag on top of that, just in case there were leaks. The tubing is pretty long and I found that I was not constrained by the bag or tubing.

The first night at home I was a bit apprehensive about what to expect, as was my wife. Again, I tried to keep myself up as long as possible, thinking I would then just crash. I worried about the bag filling, or if there would be problems with the tube. The first night I tossed and turned a bit, but essentially slept till seven in the morning.

What surprised me was that the 2 liter bag was pretty much filled! My reaction was WOW, and if this was normal, I could not imagine ever being able to sleep through the night without the catheter. My bladder would not be big enough!

What I found was that sleeping was not a problem. After the first night, I really pretty much slept through the night and had no issues or problems. After a night or so, it became completely routine. Go upstairs, drain the leg bag; put on the big bag; make my little nest in the recliner, and go to sleep.

Part of my morning routine was to empty my bag. One morning I noticed, both in my urine and in the tubing, little tiny blood clots. At first this kind of alarmed me, but the key was that the lines seemed to continue to drain. The bags continued to fill. So there was no obvious blockage or problem. If your doctor did not mention that you might see little clots, don't panic, but if anything seems out of the ordinary, call the doctor on call. They don't charge by the call or by the hour -- it is for the job!!! So don't hesitate if you are concerned over any issue.

Surprisingly, I assumed that after the catheter was out, I would just plop into my own bed and resume life as usual. This did not quite happen for me. After the catheter was removed -- remember it may be only eight days after you have had major surgery -- I found I continued to be more comfortable sleeping in my recliner, so I did. The message here is this – there is no time table as to when or how you are to sleep.

Also, when I did get back into my own bed, I found that I could only sleep on my back and with some pillows under my head and shoulder. When I tried to role a bit more toward my side, I found it uncomfortable. Now oddly enough, one night I decided to try to see what would happen if I tried sleeping on my stomach. Much to my surprise, it was quite comfortable. However, the problem I found was getting there, i.e. rolling over. After lying for some time on my stomach, I found my neck was stressed from having my head turned to the side for a long period of time. So, I accepted sleeping on my back was good enough. It was some weeks before I could begin to feel comfortable on my side or partially on my side. Somewhere between four and six weeks, I began to feel pretty normal again. All of a sudden I realized that I didn't have an ache or a pain, or was comfortable in different positions.

Also, remember, you are not going to have your normal energy and stamina. Milk it for all its worth! Lie around, watch TV, rent movies, walk in the yard, or read the paper from cover to cover. Look at your wife, kids, or whomever you can get sympathy from and ask them if they would mind getting you a nibble or two! Leave work early and come in late: hey, you gotta get some enjoyment out of this!

In all seriousness, I was not back up to speed for a good month, but that didn't mean I could not do anything. My wife and I went to a movie and out for something to eat the night after my catheter was out, just 9 days after surgery! I just walked slower. I also did not have my old energy level and I found myself wanting to take a nap at times.

Chapter 7.

BM's

Prune juice, hemorrhoids and other fun things.

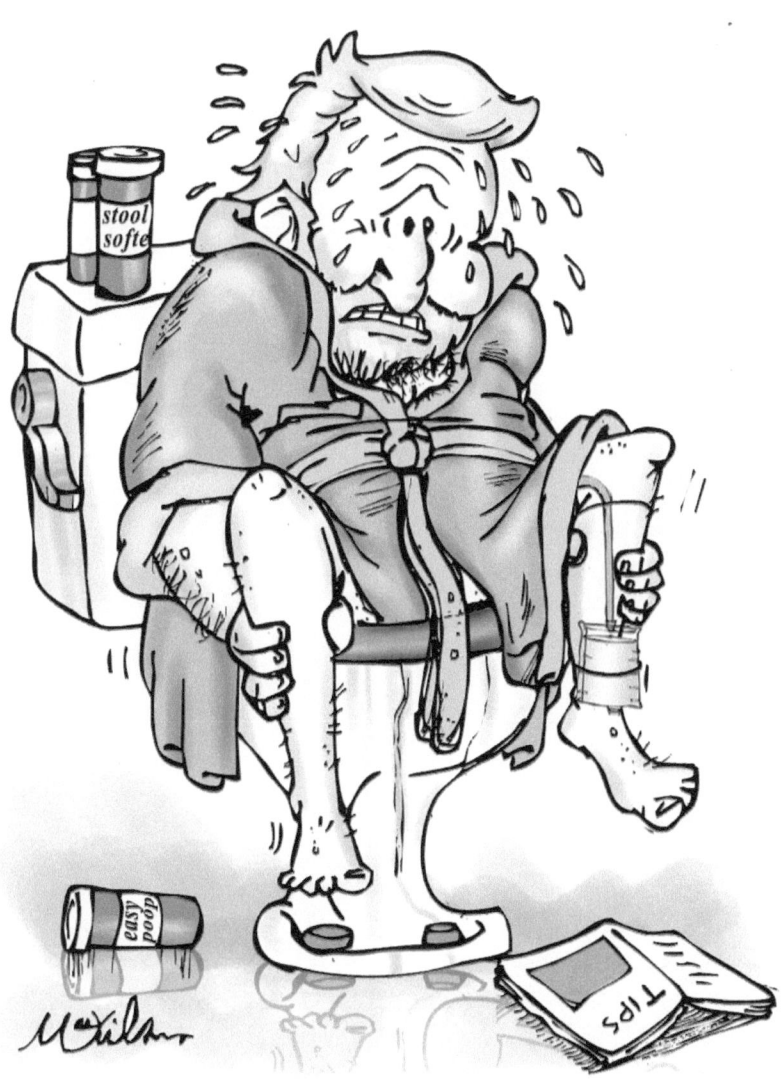

I hate to get back to bodily functions again, but, the first big bench mark is getting out of bed. Next is walking. Then passing gas and eating. The last item is having a BM.

Remember, prior to surgery, I got totally cleaned out. I did not really eat for a day or two. So I didn't have much in the old pipeline! I had my surgery on Thursday afternoon. On Friday my doctor told me I could go home and not to expect to have a BM till Monday. In the meantime, he gave me a combo pill to take, a stool softener and laxative together in one little brown pill. You can buy these little beauties over the counter and they are generic. Ask the pharmacist for them.

Well, the good doctor knew what he was talking about. On Monday afternoon, it happened and it was no big deal. I continued to take a stool softener (without the laxative) for the balance of the week.

A couple of issues here for me. First, for a number of weeks after my surgery, going to the bathroom was never a problem, but it felt different. I am not sure if I can describe it, but if you remember back to when you had your biopsy and afterward the "discomfort" you may have felt in your colon/rectum, it was similar to this. It did not really reach the level of what I would call pain, but it was not business as usual. It is like your colon is sore or bruised.

This was further complicated by hemorrhoids. Now I realize that this will probably not happen to most people. In case it does, it did not present a problem, just a factor to deal with along with some discomfort. So my caution here is this. If you have had hemorrhoids, or are prone to them, be a good boy scout and be prepared with hemorrhoid cream, or whatever you find is helpful for you.

I would suggest baby wipes as well. You are going to be doing a lot of sitting and lying around which may factor into all this. Prior to the surgery, I did a bit of planning as to where in the house I was going to be spending my time, ensuring that I had easy access to a bathroom.

I found that after the catheter was out I wanted to go to the bathroom much more frequently. As my bladder filled, I had a different kind of sensation then I have ever had in the past. It is not a painful one, but if you are anything like me, you are going to notice that there is a pressure in and around your bladder and I have to assume it is the pressure of the bladder filling and pushing/straining against the sutures holding things together inside me (I assume where the two ends of the urethra are joined). Also, I was concerned over bladder control and anxious to get rid of my diapers.

DIAPERS: prior to surgery, I had this notion of what this was going to be like. Well, I have some good news: it is not a big deal and not uncomfortable. The *Depends* are like wearing briefs, just a bit bulkier. The issue I had was more with the "imploding" feeling I mentioned earlier. When I sat, I assume the pants get pushed a bit more against your body and this pushes on your penis as well. It just kind of feels a little different and will take a bit of getting used to.

I was extremely lucky in that my wearing of *Depends* really only lasted a day and a half. That does not mean that I was 100% like I was before surgery. What I found was this: I had almost 100% control over what I will call normal bladder function. I could hold it in, release it on demand, and for the most part prevent drips or leaks.

BUT there is one exception. When I passed gas, I found that when I relaxed one sphincter (rectum) my bladder sphincter also relaxed; this was sometimes a challenge. So I found that I did not force or cause myself to pass gas if I could help it. The big exception to this is when I was actually going to the bathroom (urinating). Then, I did not have to worry about this at all and I could be as relaxed as I wanted, so to speak! Your friends and loved ones will appreciate this new dynamic!

I found that it was almost a full six weeks after surgery before I really felt "normal." And even then it wasn't totally like it was. I had an "awareness" of my bodily functions that was somewhat different. I imagined it would just take time. And I was right.

Chapter 8.

Walking and exercising

You ain't broke, get over it.

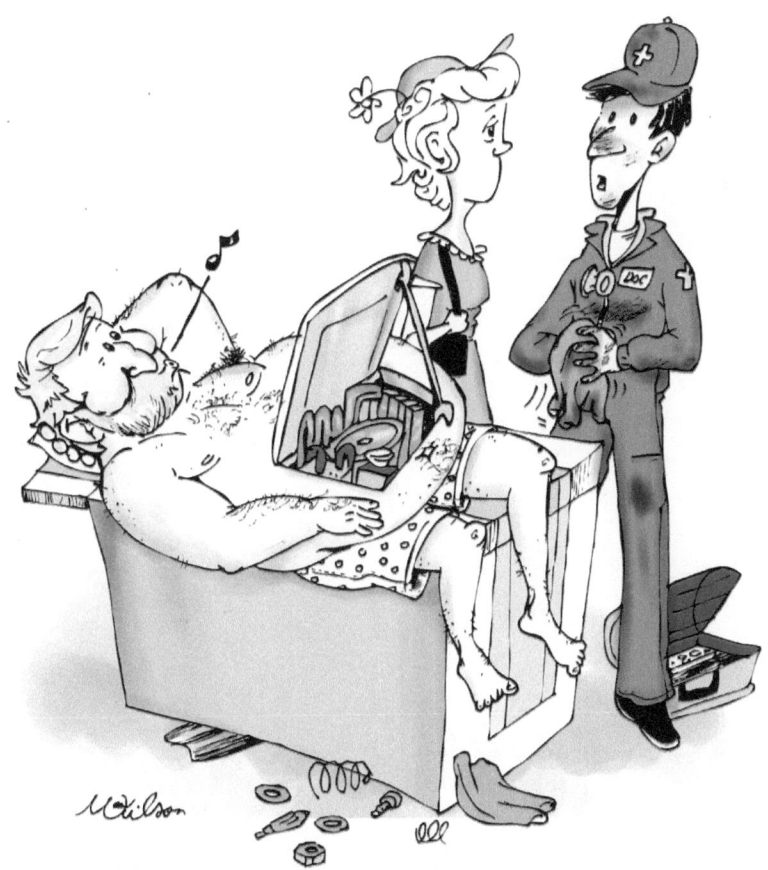

"Everything seems to check out alright...only thing I can recommend is exercise, get his motor goin' and to tell your husband if it aint broke...get over it."

I began writing this little handbook immediately after surgery. It is now almost three months since. I mention this because I find it amazing that in that short time how much I have already forgotten about my experience, which is a good sign, right?

Walking is one of the major elements to the recovery process. It begins the day after surgery. That first walk was a bit of a challenge – more from anticipated fear than from anything else. But if you are like me, you will be motivated to walk for two reasons. First, you ain't going home if you can't walk! Second, what are your other options: sitting in a chair or lying in bed? Neither of these was particularly appealing to me. So I walked, and you will, too.

Walking does a number of things. It gets your body functions moving, literally. They don't call it a bowel movement for nothing. Walking jiggles your insides and helps get the gas in motion and, trust me, you want motion.

Walking also kills time. At first I found that I did not have much of an interest in reading – or rather sitting and concentrating, which is kind of necessary to read. Have you ever watched old movies where the guy in jail paces his cell over and over again and knows just how many paces there are from wall to wall? Well, at the time, I could have told you the exact number of steps from one bedroom to another. The reality is that I needed the exercise, so although walking the same paths became boring, it was doing my body good.

I am assuming that most men who have this operation are going to be 50+ and probably more like 60+. Well, welcome to the world of aging! One of the characteristics I have found with my friends and me is the rapid degeneration of our bodies and muscles.

So not only did I walk, I also developed a little exercise routine. It consisted of slight knee bends, stretches, getting up on my toes, and what I called countertop pushups. For these, I went into the kitchen, stood a few feet away from the countertop, leaned forward, and did little pushups. I think part of the value of this drill is not just for the exercising itself, but also for the psychological reinforcement that you are not broken.

Now all this said, the reality is that you are not going to have a great deal of energy after the operation for some weeks to come. So you have to use your head a bit and not overdo it while at the same time not becoming a couch potato.

There is another entirely different aspect to exercising that I also want to address. Your doctor will talk to you about doing kegel exercises. Below is a Wikipedia listing you can check out (isn't Wikipedia amazing?): (**http://en.wikipedia.org/wiki/ Kegel_exercise).**

Now I have absolutely no empirical proof of what I am about to say, so take it for what it is worth. A few days after I came home with my catheter, I kind of wondered about the whole dynamic of urinating. In fact one of the questions I have been asked is will you know when you are urinating when you have a catheter in? And the answer is no.

I began wondering if I was going to be able to control my bladder output once the catheter was out. So I experimented a bit with trying to "use" my muscles as I would normally when going to the bathroom, i.e. being able to start and stop peeing. Of course with the catheter in I could not start and stop. But I could "flex" my muscles just like I was starting and stopping.

What this told me was, a) I could feel my muscles, which meant that the nerves going to them must be ok; and b) I could very easily do those things that normally would start and stop my peeing. I extended this little exercising to kegel exercises, even though my catheter was in. I am convinced that this exercising contributed to my being able to have bladder control almost instantly post surgery. I got rid of my *Depends* a day and a half after the catheter was removed and have had virtually no issue of leaking or dripping.

So my advice is this: exercise both in the normal modes like walking, leg stretches, and arm and body exercises. AND, do Kegel exercises almost from the get go. Don't wait till the catheter is out. And, of course, don't overdo it and be sensitive to your body.

All in all, when it was all "over" I lost about eight pounds. Unfortunately, I have since found most of them – they were hiding in the refrigerator!

Chapter 9.

Breathing, coughing and sneezing

Oh my god!

In the hospital the nurses gave me a little breathing gadget. I found when they first gave it to me that I could barely move the little balls up the tube. In fact, I was sure that this thing was not functioning properly. Then my son came to visit, picked it up and made the balls go to the top of the tube and stay there for almost a full minute.

This was great for me for a couple of reasons. First, it showed that it could be done. Second, there was no way in hell that I was going to let my son make me look like an old man that could not even make the little balls go up to the top of the tube. In reality, this is a critical exercise not only for your lungs, but for your abdominal muscles.

Your abdominal wall is going to feel like you have been slapped a thousand times. It is going to be sore; you are not going to want to be doing sit ups. I found after a few days of working with this little devil I made great progress and realized that I wasn't broken. I could make my muscles work and do what I needed them do.

Sneezing and coughing are awful. I immediately came to this conclusion after the first sneeze and cough and did not want to do it a second time.

Sneezing is the worse. Just for kicks, I again went to Wikipedia and darn if I didn't find a whole listing on sneezing – who puts this stuff in there and is there nothing that is not listed? Anyway, as you know *"the sneeze reflex is an involuntary, sudden, violent, and audible expulsion of air through the mouth and nose."* The key here is the involuntary, sudden, and violent characteristics.

I am not sure what to tell you here, other than to have some level of cognizance that this may happen. My advice is to try to close it down as much as possible. But when all is said and done, you won't break.

Chapter 10.

A Really important subject…

Your wife, partner, caretaker, children and friends

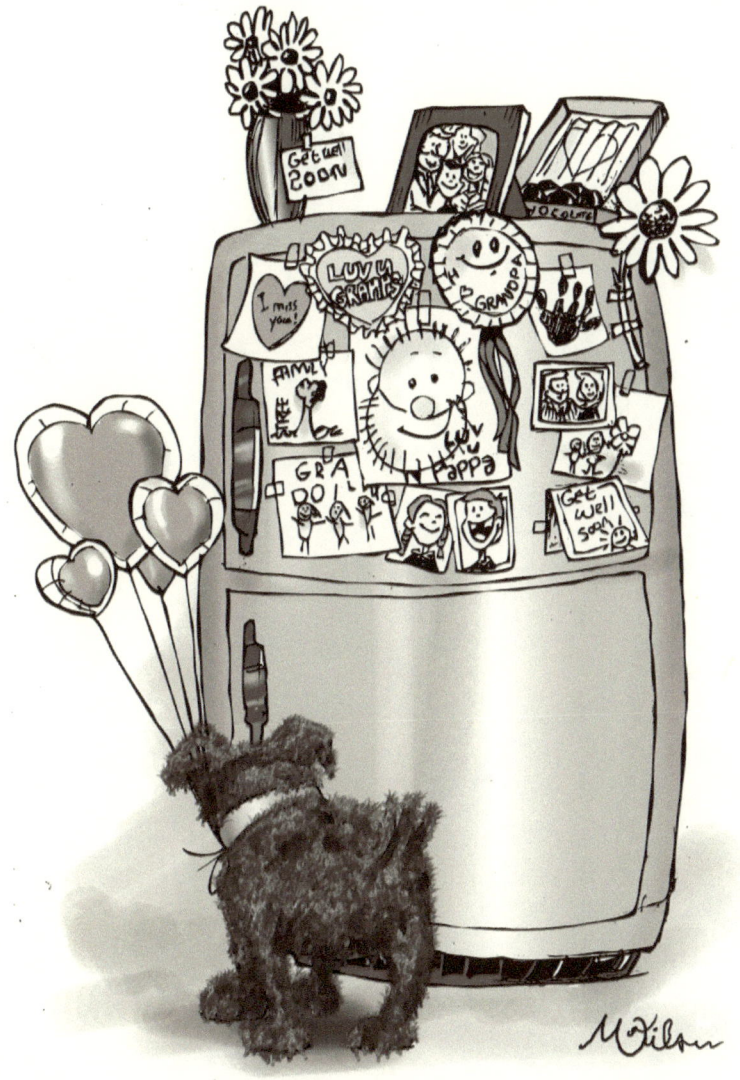

Well, I have really covered most of the physical issues that I dealt with post surgery. There is another topic, however, that I do feel worth addressing, and that deals with all the people in your world.

The first thing you are going to have to address is who to tell and how. Now being a person with a real gallows humor, my immediate thoughts were, there must be a way to get some fun and/or shock value out of all this. So I dreamed up all kinds of ways to tell people, like, "Hey, did I happen to mention that I have cancer?" I figured I might as well have some enjoyment with it.

I found out very quickly that probably was not the best way to let people know. Then I went almost 180 degrees in the opposite direction and began worrying about telling people because they just don't know how to react. And then again, there is cancer and there is CANCER. With a little luck I was going to be able to claim survivor status without a lot of trauma and stress. So when I told people, in the same breath I said something to the effect that I was going to have my prostate removed but that it appeared to be in the very early stages and I was not overly concerned. Be prepared because they will then tell you, in reassuring terms, of all the friends, neighbors and relatives that have had prostate cancer and all are doing very well.

The reality is that in some ways having cancer and prostate surgery was more traumatic for my family than it was for me. This was evidenced immediately after surgery when I was taken to my room and my wife and son were there all smiley and happy because they had been told how successful the operation was. I was not nearly as happy and smiley! But for them, the first and scariest part of the process was over. For me, the worst part was just beginning. I have never had any health issues prior to this so I guess I had always maintained my role as DAD... which means a lot of different things to different family members, but the one thing it probably does not normally convey is weakness and fragility.

I remember one of the things my son said when I first got to the room and was in my bed. He was looking down on me, and said, "Boy you look a lot smaller." That really hit me because I remember when my dad was hospitalized and I saw him lying in bed, weakened and ill, and thinking how small and fragile the old lion seemed.

I share this because they are going to be as scared as you, if not more so. I was surprised at how upset my wife was and how one day my daughter just looked at me and started to cry and, of course, then so did I.

Speaking of crying, I observed something I thought interesting about my own emotionality. Again, I have no empirical data to support this and have no idea if it is related or not. I have found that I am much more emotional than I was before the surgery. I know when my wife had bypass surgery a number of years ago one of the surprising side effects was extreme emotionality and particularly fear of being left alone. So for what it is worth, I mention it.

One more element of having cancer and surgery is that you are going to find, if you aren't already aware of it, that you have more friends and neighbors than you can imagine that either have had prostate cancer, or are in the process of having this same experience. I found it very helpful to talk to them. As I said in the beginning of this little booklet, that men don't generally talk about substantive stuff like this. I found it really helpful talking to others, but this is a very individualistic experience. Yours will not be like mine or anyone else's for that matter. But there will be a lot of shared experiences as well and I found it helpful talking to friends. I did find that it was me that had to initiate that conversation, as is customary because most people don't like to bring up someone else's cancer. I say, don't hesitate to talk about it!

Chapter 11.

Hell, that wasn't so bad!

It's out? Now what?

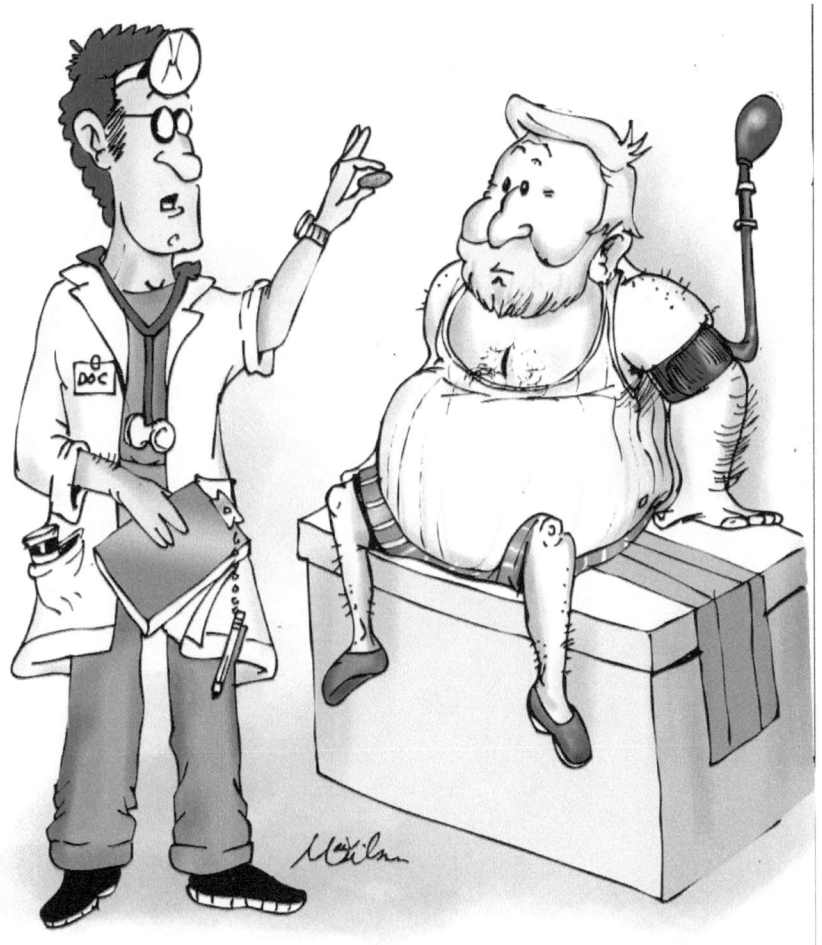

"You are going to love this pill."

Well it has been almost three months since my surgery. I am more or less back to my old self, with some very distinct exceptions.

The two big "concerns" of prostate surgery (even "successful" surgery) are the issue of incontinence and impedance.

For me the incontinence was virtually a non-issue. However, I can still sense some bodily changes and feelings. I am not concerned and they don't really present any challenges to me – just a simple awareness that things are a bit different now. I also suspect that this will continue to change and become less and less noticeable as time goes by.

Each medical practice will handle the entire process, including the part about impotence counseling, differently. On the day I had my catheter removed, my doctor told me that I would have an appointment in a month with their erection specialist. To be candid, I envisioned a large buxom young blonde. I was most curious about meeting her as well as discussing her treatment plan! Alas, when I made my appointment, the specialist was not a buxom young blonde. The specialist's name was David.

To be honest, I was a bit nervous and curious as to what this visit with David was going to entail. I won't even begin to spell out the variety of different things that went through my head. So, I went to my appointment as scheduled with lots of thoughts in my head, but no facts.

David turned out to be a very nice gentleman with a warm smile and sense of humor, and he was not much younger than me. I went into the examination room and there on the walls and counter were an assortment of anatomical drawings of the male genitalia as well as some very interesting apparatus.

Well it turned out that David's primary function seemed to be to tell me what some of my options were in terms of getting an erection. They ranged from pills to a gizmo that looked like a big plastic tube that created a vacuum (you can use your own imagination). One option involved injections. I know, the thought of injecting your penis is a bit difficult to imagine, but I did have him do it just so I could determine my options. It was not painful, and it works almost instantly, but I decided I would pass on this.

My doctor also prescribed a daily low dose of Cialis to help the healing process. Here I need to give you a cautionary note about my Cialis experience. About a month after the surgery, while taking a daily lose dose of Cialis, I began having heartburn. It became bothersome enough that I went to see a gastroenterologist who did an endoscopy. Much to my amazement, I did some research and I informed the gastroenterologist that in 0-10% of men taking low dose Cialis develop gastric problems. He was not aware of this. I quit taking it, and was almost instantly better.

Now back to erections. It turns out that there is a "use it or lose it" aspect to erections. But the most important thing he told me was that this could be an 18 month long process and don't expect too much too quickly.

This kind of surprised me because I just assumed that if the blood vessels and nerves were not cut, then they would just work. This turns out not to be the case. In talking to a friend of mine about this he made some comments that I didn't fully get, but am beginning to understand. He had his (traditional – non-robotic) surgery about a year and a half ago. In cheering me on, he made a comment about how things are working but not quite the same as the good old days. Heck, that was true prior to the surgery too! He talked about the need for he and his wife to be a bit more creative now. To be honest I didn't explore this at the time, and may have to go back to find out more.

The key is this. I am alive, in good health, and have very little concern that my prostate cancer is going to be life threatening. So everything else becomes simply an issue to deal with and adjust to. When all is said and done, for me this is not an issue of concern.

So good luck! You will find that in no time you will be back in the game and enjoying life to its fullest.

Harvey Silver

Appendix:

A. Shared experiences from other patients.

It is my hope that others who go through this experience will be willing to share their own unique experience so others can benefit from it as well.

- If you are so inclined to do so, please send them to me at:

  harveysilver@me.com

- I have created a blog for sharing experiences. It is:

  www.myprostatecancer101.com

- Tower Urology:

  http://www.towerurology.com/

B. Prostate Cancer Support Groups:

http://www.ustoo.com/

http://www.yananow.net/

C. Quick Facts

- The prostate gland, which is about the size of a walnut, contains cells that make some of the seminal fluid that protects and nourishes the sperm.

- There will be approximately 234,460 new cases of prostate cancer diagnosed in the United States in 2006. About 27,350 men will die of the disease this year.

- Prostate cancer is the third leading cause of cancer death in men, exceeded only by lung and colon and rectal cancer.

- Surgery offers an excellent chance for cure from cancer of the prostate.

Source: James Buchanan Brady Urological Institute

D. Two Years Later...

I had my two-year check up. My doctor said I could be the poster boy for prostate cancer! I just re-read this and was amazed at how much I had forgotten about the experience. This is a very good thing.

I feel great. I am trying to exercise regularly. And for all practical purposed, "all systems" work. In the two years I have had more friends diagnosed with prostate cancer. Some had other issues, such as diabetes and heart related issues as well. But the key data is this: all are fine and enjoying life!